The Complete Natural Beauty Secrets Guide

Homemade Beauty Products and Home Remedies for Fabulous Hair, Skin & Beauty

SCARLETT O'MARA

Table of Contents

Introduction

I want to thank you and congratulate you for purchasing this book!

This book contains proven steps and strategies on how to make your own beauty products at home.

Beauty products are some of the most expensive products on the market. Their promises of glowing and smooth skin, finer lines or no wrinkles, and unblemished and even appearance all make them desirable to millions of people all over the world. Of course, looking beautiful on the outside is ideal, but what is more important is that we take care of our bodies also from within. With this in mind, we try to look past all the labels and all the promises, and simply focus on what is truly best for our body and our health. This book will teach you how to make your own beauty products using only natural ingredients that you can find at home. By using such ingredients, you will save a lot, and you can be sure that you are giving only the best to your body.

Thanks again for purchasing this book, I hope you enjoy it! Please take some time to stop by and LIKE our Facebook page:

https://www.facebook.com/joypublishing

With gratitude,

Scarlett O'Mara

Chapter 1: Look Good, Feel Good!

People always say that beauty comes from within and that we should never judge others by their appearance, but who can deny the appeal of clear, glowing skin and soft, silky hair? Many of us want to look good because it is how we are able to feel good. When others see how well we take care of our bodies and compliment us on how good we look, there is a genuine feeling of joy and happiness that makes us look even more beautiful. After all, the only way we can project ourselves to be beautiful is when we truly feel good about ourselves.

While having a positive outlook in life, sharing good principles, and keeping healthy relationship can definitely keep us happy, it is hard to deny the fact that the body changes as we grow older. Dark spots develop on the skin, lines appear on the face, and even the hair gets damaged and turns into one big mess. Growing old may be part of growing up, but it does not mean that we have to surrender to the signs of aging that slowly take over the body. After all, many of the damages that happen to the body are caused by dirt and other irritants that a healthy body should not be exposed to.

Most of us are ashamed of these unhealthy signs. We hide the pimples and the blemishes, we try to conceal the dark spots and the rings around our eyes, and we cover up just so people will be blind to the other things that we do not want them to see. Even the hair gets special treatments so that it retains its natural shine and softness.

The beauty solutions and beauty products that we have nowadays offer a myriad of benefits. Glowing, youthful skin, bright eyes, an even skin tone, smoothness of the face and lack of blemishes and marks, and even softer hair, are now possible with the help of all these beauty products. Unfortunately, as valuable as their benefits are, they can also be quite expensive on the budget. A single-use facial mask can cost as much as $10, while special facial creams and serums are often worth hundreds of dollars each.

Luckily, many of these products are actually made from natural and organic resources that you can find in your own home. If you do not have them already, you will be happy to find that many of the ingredients you will need to make your own beauty products are easily available. You can find natural ingredients at the nearest stores or local market, or you can go to a specialty organic store for the things you need. Being healthy and beautiful is truly priceless, and you no longer have to pay too much just to enjoy such benefits.

Chapter 2: Natural Hair Treatments

The hair is one of a person's greatest assets, but it is also one that is most exposed to the harms and damages of everyday stress. Did you know that with a few kitchen essentials you can keep your hair feeling soft and naturally healthy? Eggs, honey, and yogurt are just some of the ingredients that you can use to treat your hair, and the good news is that they are more natural and less expensive than any hair product available in the market.

The Egg Wash

Raw eggs can do wonders for the hair. Yolks are rich in fats and proteins that help keep your hair moisturized. As for the egg whites, they contain bacteria-eating enzymes that can rid the hair of unwanted dirt and oil. For a simple hair treatment, all you need is one raw egg.

Those who have oily hair can use the egg white to cleanse the hair of unwanted oils, while those with dry and frizzled hair can use the yolk to moisturize hair. For those with normal hair, the whole egg can be used without any problems. Start with half a cup of the egg ingredient that you need and carefully apply to clean and damp hair. Make sure to cover the scalp and the hair so add more egg if necessary. Leave the egg treatment on for 20 minutes then wash away with cold water. Do not use hot water as this could 'cook' the egg. After rinsing off the egg, shampoo the hair and dry carefully. Treatments using whole eggs or egg yolks only can be used once a month while those making use of egg whites can be done twice a month.

Yogurt Hair Treatment

Hair can often become dull and dry because of the pollution and chemical products that it is exposed to everyday. To keep your hair staying moist and clean, use a simple yogurt treatment for your hair. The lactic acid content of yogurt cleans hair of dirt, white the milk helps moisturize your hair.

Use half a cup of plain yogurt or sour cream and massage it onto damp hair. Let it sit for 20 minutes, after which clean off with warm water. Follow up with some cold water and wash with your regular shampoo. You can do this treatment after every other week.

Itchy Scalp Treatment

Flakes brought about by stress, poor diet, and bad weather conditions can leave your scalp dry and itchy. Instead of trying a dozen anti-dandruff solutions, go natural with some olive oil and lemon juice. The lemon juice gets rid of the loose and dry flakes on your hair, and the olive oil brings back moisture to the hair.

Make a mixture by combining equal parts lemon juice to equal part olive oil and water. Start with half a tablespoon of each and combine thoroughly before massaging onto dry scalp. Leave the treatment on for 20 minutes, afterwards rinse and wash your hair with shampoo. You can do this treatment every other week.

For Dry and Sun-Damaged Hair

The sun can cause harsh damage to the hair and can cause it to be dry and brittle. The same effect also comes from treatments that involve heat, such as flat irons and curlers. If you want to treat dry and sun-damaged hair, look no further than your cupboard and reach for a bottle of honey. Honey naturally attracts and keeps in moistness, and can easily fix dry and damaged hair.

Start by using one-half cup of honey and massage it onto damp and clean hair. If you feel that the honey alone is too thick, add 1 to 2 tablespoons of olive oil. Leave it on for 20 minutes and rinse with warm water afterwards. You can also add an egg yolk or another protein-rich ingredient for severely sun-damaged hair. You can enjoy this treatment once every month.

Grape Seed Treatment

Much like honey, grape seed is great for keeping your hair and your scalp moisturized. Simply apply grape seed oil onto your hair and scalp and leave it on for about fifteen minutes. You can then wash off your hair with regular shampoo and rinse properly.

Shea Butter

Shea butter is not just a great ingredient for body lotions; it is also excellent for the hair. Apply shea butter to damaged hair by massaging onto hair and scalp. Let it rest for fifteen minutes and rinse off with warm water. The shea butter acts as a conditioner and restores life to damaged hair. It is rich in vitamins A, E, and F which is great for moisture and for mending split ends.

Olive Oil

Another natural treatment that you can use for damaged hair is extra virgin olive oil. Using extra virgin olive oil on your hair allows it to renew its strength and natural shine. The vitamin E and antioxidants that extra virgin olive oil provides also keep hair moisturized from the scalp to the tips.

Aloe Vera

Everyone knows that aloe vera has wonderful effects on hair. It has excellent moisturizing properties, and also conditions hair to keep it strong and revitalized. In some cases, aloe vera is even used to strengthen hair and to help it grow long and beautiful. If you have the plant available, simply cut a piece open and rub directly onto the scalp. This is an excellent all-natural treatment for repairing dry and damaged hair.

Coconut Milk

If you think that coconut milk is just for those yummy recipes, think again. This tropical wonder can bring great benefits to your hair. Apply it on your hair and scalp and let it rest for fifteen minutes. Rinse with warm water afterwards. Doing so will help nourish your hair as the coconut milk contains protein, fatty acids, and iron, which are all great for taking care of damaged and brittle hair with split ends.

For Greasy Hair

Sometimes, you never know what to do with the cornstarch or cornmeal that you have in the pantry. If you have this ingredient lying around, use it on your hair and you will see that it can do wonders for greasy hair.

You will need 1 tablespoon of cornstarch or cornmeal and a salt or pepper shaker. Place the cornmeal/cornstarch in the shaker and sprinkle onto dry hair and scalp. Leave it on for 10minutes then carefully brush it out with a paddle brush. You can do this as often as every other day.

For Frizzy Hair

Avocados are regularly used in beauty and health products, and it is not surprising why. The oils and proteins from the fruit provide nutrients and nourishments. With frizzy hair, the avocado can smoothen out and weigh down those errant strands.

Use half of an avocado and mash the fruit so that you can apply it to your clean, damp hair. Once the scalp and hair have been covered, let it stand for 15minutes. You can then rinse with water and wash if necessary. For added moisturizing effect, you can use a tablespoon or two of sour cream or mayonnaise. Use this treatment every two weeks and keep your hair healthy and moisturized.

For Residue-Ridden Hair

Dirt, pollution, and all the products you put into your hair develop a residue buildup that can damage it greatly. If you want to get rid of all that residue and buildup, you can use a very simple kitchen ingredient: baking soda. Baking soda cleans product buildup better than anything else.

Combine 1 to 2 tablespoons of baking soda with little amounts of water until it takes on a paste-like consistency. Apply the paste onto your scalp and hair and let sit for 15minutes. Afterwards, rinse with water and wash with shampoo. You can do this treatment once every two weeks.

For Shiny Hair

Mixing your regular conditioner with a little bit of honey can produce great results. Simply modify your conditioner by adding two to three tablespoons of honey for every cup of conditioner and use this solution after washing your hair with shampoo. Leave it on for 30minutes to let your hair have that amazing shine and softness.

Apple Cider Wash

Even apple cider can be used on the hair for a homemade treatment. Combine equal parts warm water and apple cider and apply to your hair. Wash and rinse after five minutes and make sure to get rid of the smell. This will give you naturally bouncy hair.

Almond Oil

Almond oil is another natural ingredient that you can use for your hair. Simply heat some almond oil in the microwave for about forty seconds. Apply this evenly to your hair and leave on for half an hour. Wash as you normally would with shampoo and conditioner afterwards. The almond oil strengthens your hair and repairs damages as well.

Lemon Shine

Another way to get rid of dull hair is by using some lemon juice. After washing, simply apply a tablespoon of lemon juice onto your hair. There is no need to rinse this off as you simply need to dry off and style as you normally would.

Beer Wash

A simple ingredient such as beer can be used for a home hair treatment. Before washing, pour beer evenly onto your hair and scalp. Leave this on for about twenty minutes; wash thoroughly afterwards to get rid of the smell. You can do this once a week to get soft and smooth hair.

Homemade Conditioner

Here is a simple homemade conditioner that you can make with simple ingredients from your home. To make this, combine equal parts egg and yogurt and mix until you have a uniform mixture. Rub this onto your scalp using your fingertips and leave for about five to ten minutes.

Natural Homemade Shampoo

Shampoo is a basic necessity for hair care. It cleans the scalp and hair strands, keeping it healthy and free from damage. Unfortunately, most commercial shampoos are made with chemicals that can also cause damage to the hair. If you want an all-natural product, here is a simple shampoo recipe that you could try for yourself.

Ingredients:

- ¼ cup Coconut Milk – homemade, not canned
- 1/3 cup Liquid Castille Soap
- 1 tablespoon Essential Oils of Choice – peppermint, lavender, rosemary, etc.
- ½ teaspoon Vitamin E Oil – optional
- 1/2 teaspoon Olive or Almond Oil – for dry hair

Procedure:

1. Put together all ingredients in an old shampoo bottle or in a liquid soap dispenser.

2. Combine all ingredients by shaking thoroughly.

3. Shake well before every use.

4. Keep for up to 1 month in the shower.

5. Making your own natural and homemade shampoo is easy and quick to do. You can even select the scents that you want and add vitamins and other oils that you prefer.

Homemade Hair Gel

Here is a recipe for hair gel that you can do at home. All you need are water, some flax seeds, and tools from the kitchen.

Ingredients:

- 1 cup water
- ¼ cup Flax Seeds (linseeds in UK)
- You will need: 1 large saucepan, a strainer, one large bowl, small wire whisk, 4-5 oz bottle for storing your finished product.

Procedure:

1. Pour the water into the large saucepan.

2. Add the flax seeds to the water and turn on the heat to high.

3. Stir occasionally to keep the seeds moving and to keep them from sticking to the bottom of the pan.

4. When the water comes to a full boil, stir gently and constantly. You will see a thin film of gel develop on the surface of the water.

5. Once you see the film of gel, lower the heat and continue stirring. Be sure to watch the seeds carefully and look out for when the seeds suspend in the middle of the clear gel substance instead of settling at the bottom of the pan.

6. Turn off the heat once you see the seeds being suspended. Stir one last time and pour over the strainer. Have the bowl ready below the strainer to collect the gel.

7. The gel will strain slowly so in the meantime, rinse your pan to keep the gel from getting harder.

8. If you want a thicker consistency, return the gel to the clean pan for a second time and strain once again. You can also add oils, fragrances, or other extracts by simply pouring over the gel and stirring with a whisk.

9. Transfer to the bottle and use when needed.

Chapter 3: Homemade Skin & Facial Products

Skincare products are some of the most popular in the line of beauty products that are being sold in the market today. Everyone wants to look young and fresh, and it is through beautiful and clear skin that one is able to show off a healthy disposition. However, not all skincare products are actually good for the skin. There are so many ingredients and chemicals being used in the products that you can never be sure if they are truly good for you. With this in mind, many skin care experts are turning back to all-natural products. They are safer, oftentimes much more effective, and they also help the local and small-time entrepreneurs who produce organic and all-natural goods. You can also enjoy the benefits of these natural skincare products with just a fraction of the price you would need to spend on their commercial counterparts. All you need are some kitchen ingredients and tools, and a few tips from the experts.

Oatmeal and Onion Puree Face Mask

Did you know that onions and oatmeal have surprisingly great effects on the skin? These two ingredients can do wonders for your skin, and they can be sitting and waiting to be used right at your pantry. Oatmeal is a natural cleanser and scrub that can help to clear those clogged pores. As for onions, they have natural anti-inflammatory effects that can help ease the impact of acne on your skin. Here is how you can use oatmeal and onions for an all-natural face mask.

Ingredients:

- ¼ cup Water
- 1/3 cup Plain Oatmeal
- 1 large White Onion
- 1/2 teaspoon Honey – optional

Procedure:

1. Bring the water to a boil and pour over plain oatmeal.

2. Wait for 5minutes to let the mixture steep.

3. Meanwhile, puree the onion in a food processor until you have a smooth paste-like substance.

4. Add the pureed onion to the oatmeal while it is still warm. You can also add honey at this point to let the mixture have a thicker consistency.

5. Stir the mixture until well combined.

6. Spread on the face, making sure to be careful around the eyes, the nose, and the lips. Let sit for 10 minutes. You can

adjust the consistency of the mask by adding more honey to the mixture if necessary.

7. Rinse off with cold water.

8. The oatmeal-onion mixture should be able to keep well for one week. Be sure to keep it in the refrigerator for proper storage. Simply warm up a bit before using on the face, and remember not to place it in the freezer as doing so can ruin the mixture.

Homemade Coffee Mask

Coffee is an absolute staple for millions of people all over the world. Aside from being one of the most popular drinks today, it is also one of the best ingredients that go into beauty and skincare products. Scrubs and facial cleansers have been developed using the magic of coffee, and now you can make your own homemade coffee mask as well.

Ingredients:

- 3 tablespoons Ground Coffee – fine; used
- 1 cup Milk

Procedure:

1. Place the ground coffee in a bowl. You can even use the ground coffee that you used for your morning drink.

2. Slowly pour the milk over the coffee and stir properly to get it thoroughly mixed. Add only a little at a time until you achieve a thick consistency just enough that you will be able to put it onto your face and it won't drip off. If the mixture becomes too runny or wet, simply add more ground coffee. So, make sure that you have a little bit left on the side as well.

3. When ready to use, apply the coffee and milk mixture onto your face by smoothening it out carefully. Be sure to avoid the eyes and the lips.

4. Massage the paste onto your face slowly and let it sit for 20minutes as you relax.

5. Rinse off with water while continuing to massage the mixture onto your face. The coffee will also act as an exfoliating scrub at this point.

6. Pat your face dry with a clean towel and apply moisturizer while your skin is still damp to seal in the moisture.

7. You should feel the difference immediately and see that your skin will be smoother and softer. Also, using this coffee mask will help give that extra glow to your face.

Homemade Facial Toners

Facial toners are essential for keeping the face clean and healthy. It helps to remove unwanted impurities such as dust and dirt particles, and it helps remove excess oils as well. An effective toner is also able to tighten the pores so that they do not accumulate too many impurities. This also helps the skin tighten, thus reducing fine lines and wrinkles. If you want to make your own toners at home, here are a few do-it-yourself solutions that you can try.

Cucumber Toner

Ingredients:

- ½ Cucumber
- ½ Tomato
- ¼ cup Vodka

Procedure:

1. Slice the cucumber and tomatoes into chunks.

2. Place the chopped cucumber and tomatoes, as well as the vodka into a blender or food processor and mix all ingredients together until smooth and consistent.

3. Using your fingertips, dip into the mixture and dab onto your face.

4. Let it rest for 5 minutes.

5. Rinse off with warm water and pat your face dry with a clean towel.

6. The ingredients combine to act as astringents which will remove dirt and other impurities as well as tone the skin. Excess toner can be stored in the refrigerator while completely sealed and can be used until the next day.

Green Tea Toner

Green tea is naturally healthy and beneficial in many ways. A simple cup of green tea can be a soothing drink, or it can be used as an all-natural toner that will help clean the face and give it a natural glow.

Ingredients:

- 2 teaspoons Green Tea powder
- ½ cup Boiling Water

Procedure:

1. Steep the green tea by pouring the boiling water over the powder.

2. Let sit for 10 minutes.

3. Let it cool before applying to the skin.

4. When ready to use, apply using cotton balls. Simply dip the cotton balls into the tea and then dab onto the face.

Lemon Facial Scrub

The acidity of lemon is also great for cleaning the face and ridding the skin of dirt and dust particles. To make a simple lemon facial scrub, combine equal amounts lemon zest and powdered milk to half part lemon juice. Add two parts almond meal and combine them all together until you can rub it on your face. This treatment scrub is very fragrant and lightens the skin tone.

Strawberry Mask

For a refreshing and fruity facial treatment, get some fresh strawberries, milk, and some cornstarch. The strawberry contains antioxidants that help keep your skin feel young and fresh, and the milk allows your skin to become smooth and soft. Simply combine 2 cups of fresh strawberries, 1 tablespoon fresh milk, and 1 tablespoon cornstarch. Combine all of the ingredients until you have a smooth paste and apply to your face. Leave the strawberry mask on for twenty minutes and wash afterwards with warm water.

Carrot Facial

Carrots are great for the eyes, and are also ideal for a facial mask. Cook about two to three large carrots and mash them until you have a smooth paste. Mix this with four and a half tablespoons of honey and apply directly to your face. Let it rest for ten minutes then rinse off with cool water. Carrots are rich in vitamins A and C, which both help protect the skin from sun damage. The carrot juice also moisturizes the skin and repairs facial tissues that have been damaged or worn out.

Almond Mask

Natural products are easy to use and can often bring the most benefits. For an easy facial treatment, simply soak some almonds in milk. Do this in the morning and by night, you should be able to mash the almond pieces until you have a fine paste. You can add more milk if necessary, or you can simply use a blender or food processor to ease the procedure. Apply the paste to your face just before sleeping and leave it on for the duration of the night. Simply wash off with cold water in the morning and you will see your face become lighter and feel smoother (if you use it two times in a week).

Honey and Lemon Juice

With all the benefits of honey and lemon juice on your skin, hair, and body, you should have them already available in your pantry. For your face, mix equal parts honey and equal parts lemon juice and apply on the face. Let it rest for half an hour then rinse with warm water.

Bread Crumbs and Milk Cream

Milk is great on the skin, and so is milk cream. By mixing it with simple ingredients, even breadcrumbs, you can have fair and glowing skin after just fifteen minutes. Simply combine bread crumbs and milk cream and let the mixture rest for 2 minutes. Once it is soft enough, apply on your face like a regular face mask and leave on for 15 minutes before rinsing off with clean water.

Rice Mask

Rice can also be used with milk to make an all-natural facial scrub. Simply soak rice in milk for two hours and grind it until you have a coarse paste. Apply the scrub on the face and leave on for ten minutes. You can use this scrub every other day to get soft and glowing skin.

Watermelon Toner

If you are looking for something more summery and fresh, try this watermelon toner that will surely be able to make your skin soft and glowing.

Ingredients:

- 2 tablespoons Fresh Watermelon Juice
- 1 tablespoon Vodka
- 2 tablespoons Distilled Water

Procedure:

1. Make fresh watermelon juice by mashing half a cup or so of watermelons. Pass the mashed watermelon over a strainer or gauze to collect the juice.

2. Add a tablespoon of vodka to the watermelon juice, as well as the 2 tablespoons of distilled water.

3. Mix until well combined.

4. Apply with the use of cotton balls. Dip the cotton onto the mixture and dab onto the face.

5. Rinse with warm water.

6. You can store your watermelon toner in a glass container – tightly sealed and refrigerated. This can keep up to 10 days.

Facial Steam for Clogged Pores

The pores can easily get clogged up because of dirt and pollution, and clogged pores often lead to skin and facial problems like acne. To take care of your skin and clear up clogged pores, you can do this simple cleansing facial steam that is guaranteed to give your skin the treatment that it needs.

Ingredients:

- 1 gallon Boiling Water
- 8ml essential oils – peppermint, rosemary, lavender, etc.

Procedure:

1. Boil one gallon of water and pour over a large bowl.

2. Wait for the water to cool down a bit then add the essential oils.

3. Position your face over the bowl so that the steam is able to go directly to your skin.

4. Place a towel over your head to help keep the steam in.

5. Let the steam wash over your face for around 10 minutes.

6. Pat your face dry with a clean towel.

The steam acts to loosen the pores and flush out the unwanted impurities on the face. You can use essential oils of your choice and even mix and match a few, but keep in mind that each type of oil has its own benefits. Peppermint can be used to soothe and smooth out skin, while rosemary is a natural relaxant. Lavender is also great as it not only relaxes the muscles but also soothes and conditions the face as well as acts as an astringent to clean out impurities.

Lemon Oil Facial Peel

Of all essential oils, lemon oil is the only type that can be used directly on the face. Other types would need a carrier, namely oil, such as olive oil, Jojoba, or almond oil. Lemon is often used in beauty products and cleansers because it helps lighten skin naturally. As an exfoliating agent, lemon oil is also able to cleanse the skin of impurities and dirt.

Simply apply a few drops of lemon oil onto the face. You can use a washcloth or cotton balls to make this easier. Rub the oil onto your face and let it sit for a minute or two. Finally, rinse with cool water.

Citrus Peel and Baking Soda Scrub

Facial scrubs are highly effective for cleaning and smoothening out the skin. Scrubs contain micro beads that are able to cleanse the face of miniscule impurities and dirt particles that normal facial cleansers are not able to get rid of. Did you know that a common household product also has the same effect as these micro bead cleansers? Baking soda is made up of small particles that resemble fine micro bead cleansers. The smaller the size of the beads, the better they are as they are gentler on the skin and they are also able to reach into the smaller spaces on the face. Follow up a citrus acid peel treatment with a baking soda scrub to rid your face of impurities and to help smoothen out your skin.

For the citrus peel, combine half a cup of plain yogurt, one tablespoon of orange juice, and one tablespoon of lemon juice. Mix them all together until you have a uniform mixture, then apply onto the face with the use of your fingers. Apply the mixture onto your face using circular motions and let it stay on for 10 minutes. Finally, rinse off with some cool water.

As for the baking soda scrub, simply get some baking soda and apply to the face using your fingertips. Scrub your face with the baking soda by making small circles around your face. If you feel that the baking soda alone is too rough, mix it with a little bit of mild facial cleanser and apply to your skin. You can then rinse it off with warm water.

Apple Cider Vinegar

Anti-acne treatments are among the more popular items in facial care. If you want a simple natural remedy for acne, simply use one part pure and unfiltered apple cider vinegar and three parts fresh water. Use a cotton ball to apply the mixture to your face and leave on for at least ten minutes and up to the whole night. You can reapply it multiple times a day; just make sure to clean properly and finish off with a moisturizer.

Milk & Honey

Milk and honey are the perfect combination to keep your skin smooth, soft, and acne free. Simply combine equal parts honey and milk or yogurt. Make sure to let the temperature come to a comfortable level so that you are not surprised by the coldness of the milk or yogurt. Using a cotton pad, apply the mixture to your face. You can also simply pat it on with your fingertips. Let the mixture dry up a bit before applying another layer until you get the mask thickness that you want. Leave it on for ten to fifteen minutes then wash off with warm water. Apply moisturizer after rinsing.

Egg Whites

If you ever have some extra egg whites lying around, try using them as a facial treatment rather than throwing them away. Egg whites are perfect for fighting acne and excess oils, and they also help replenish the skin cells on your body. Simply whisk up egg whites until they are frothy then let them sit for 2 to 3 minutes. You can then apply the mixture on your face using your fingertips. Let it dry first before adding another layer until you have the thickness that you want. Finally, let the mask rest on your face for 20 minutes before rinsing with warm water. Put some moisturizer afterwards to keep your skin from drying out.

Grape Mix Cleanser

Citrus fruits, including grapes, are a natural remedy for wrinkling and aging skin. Grapes are high in antioxidants and rich in vitamins, and they also have natural exfoliating properties that help clear the skin. To make your grape anti-wrinkle cleanser, combine half a cup of grapes, a teaspoon of olive oil, one-fourth cup of yogurt, and a tablespoon of baking soda. Blend these together until you have a smooth mixture that you can apply to your face. Let it rest on your skin for five to ten minutes, then rinse off with warm water.

Grape Wash

An even simpler home treatment is to simply slice a few pieces of grapes in half and to crush them over your face. The juice and the pulp will deliver the nutrients that your skin needs, keeping your face looking young and healthy.

Milk Cleanser

Nothing can be simpler than some fresh milk to clean the face. To apply a milk cleanser, soak a face towel in some cold milk. Use the towel to apply the milk to your face, holing it in one area for about five minutes or so. Wash off with clean water and do not worry if you feel that there is still some residue left. What you feel is the lactic acid left over that actually helps exfoliate the skin.

Chapter 4: DIY Body Treatments

Getting body treatments is among the main reasons why people visit the spa. It is basically like giving your whole body a facial of some sort – after the treatment, your skin will feel soft and smooth to the touch. However, regularly going to the spa for such treatments may be hard to maintain and prove to be impractical for some. Wouldn't it be great if you just knew how to recreate them? Fortunately for you, this is something that can be done, and chances are most of the ingredients you'll need are already in your kitchen cupboard. Why bother spending so much money on expensive spa treatments when you already have the resources to make your very own skincare products within the comforts of your own home?

Sugar, pineapples, grapes, and milk are just some of the ingredients that you can work with. They are among the most effective skin care ingredients because of their high nutrient content. Keep in mind that the things you put on your skin will be absorbed effectively, so you are basically feeding your skin from the surface. An interesting fact is that you can find the aforementioned ingredients as well as their byproducts in many expensive skin care and anti-aging creams on the market today. For example, it may cost you hundreds of dollars to avail of glycolic acid peels in salons or clinics. On the other hand, one of glycolic acid's purest forms, caster sugar, is something that you can easily find and purchase at the supermarket for just $3 per bag or even less.

Are you now ready to create your own home spa recipes from the yummy ingredients in your kitchen? If so, here are some of the things that you can try out:

Apple Pie Skin Polish

Apples are well known for various nutritional benefits. They contain high amounts of vitamins A and C, potassium, and malic acid, which is an exfoliating enzyme that is effective in removing surface dirt and dead skin cells.

Ingredients:

- 2 tbsp. brown sugar
- 2 tbsp. granulated sugar
- 1 tbsp. apple sauce or fresh apple puree
- ⅛ tsp. cinnamon

Mix everything and stir well. In the bath, apply the scrub to your skin and massage in circles using bath gloves, a wash cloth, or a loofah. Concentrate on rough spots such as the elbows, knees, and heels. Rinse thoroughly and apply a rich body lotion after. Omit the granulated sugar if you plan to use it on the face. Brown sugar dissolves gently so it is more appropriate for the face's delicate skin.

Banana Sugar Body Scrub

Put bananas to home spa recipe use when you see them starting to brown. This recipe relies mostly on the banana and the sugar's skin-related benefits, but you may choose to add a little bit of oil if you wish.

Ingredients:

- A ripe banana
- 3 tbsp. granulated sugar

Optional: ¼ tsp. of your favorite essential oil or pure vanilla extract

Smash ingredients using a fork until the mixture turns thick and sticky. Be careful not to overdo it or else it will be too thin. In the bath, gently massage the mixture all over your body. If you want a banana facial scrub, set aside bananas to be mashed separately without the sugar. Avoid the eye area when scrubbing your face and rinse it off with warm water afterwards.

Pumpkin Slather

Aside from soups, pies, and Halloween decorations, pumpkins also make great body treatments.

Ingredients:

- 1 pumpkin (small)
- 1 cup yogurt
- 1 lemon

Cut the pumpkin, remove the skin, and extract the pulp. Prepare a pot of water, throw in your cut-up pumpkins, and cook until they're soft enough to be mashed. Turn off the heat, mash the pumpkin, then squeeze out the juice from the lemon and add the yogurt. Make sure that you use this mixture while it is warm. In the bath, take a seat and slather the pumpkin mixture all over your skin and let it rest for around 10 minutes. Shower with warm water afterwards. Your skin will feel nice and soft because the dead skin cells have just been removed.

Nutty Sesame Body Scrub

Sesame is among the most deeply-penetrating and soothing oils around. This recipe includes salt, and the purpose of which is to slough off dry skin. The oil, on the other hand, acts as a skin moisturizer.

Ingredients:

- 1 cup sesame seeds
- 1 cup sea salt or kosher salt
- ½ to ¾ cup sesame or sweet almond oil

Toast your sesame seeds at 350°F for around 2 minutes. The oil will be released and as a result your scrub will smell more enticing. Then, use a mortar and pestle to crush the seeds and the salt. Add the oil then gently massage the mixture on your skin, from the neck down to your toes. Or you can also do it like the pros do – from the finger and toe tips toward the heart to improve blood flow and circulation.

Lavender Milk Bath

They say that milk has great benefits for the skin, and the number of skin products available today that make use of the ingredient only proves this point. Why not make a milk bath of your own and choose the ingredients for yourself?

Ingredients:

- 1 ½ cup Whole Milk or Cream – you can also use a combination of the two
- 1/3 cup Honey
- 3 tablespoons Dried Lavender Flowers – or other dried flowers that you prefer

Start by processing the lavender flowers in a blender until they become fine powder. Transfer the lavender powder into a bowl and whisk in the milk or cream. Finally, add in the honey and mix thoroughly until well combined. Transfer into a jar for storage and before every use, make sure to shake well to incorporate all the ingredients. Use half of the mixture for one full bath to have your skin feeling smooth and refreshed. You can store the leftovers in a refrigerator for up to a week.

Almond Oil Treatment

If you want a very simple yet effective body moisturizer, all you need is all-natural almond oil. The oil is rich in vitamin E and is gentle on the skin. Simply rub some oil onto your body to retain skin elasticity. This treatment also reduces the occurrence of stretch marks so make sure to use it up to two times a day.

Hand and Foot Exfoliant

Spa treatments are never complete unless they cover the hands and the feet as well. Treat your full body well with this homemade exfoliant using only simple ingredients that you can find at home.

Ingredients:

- 8-10 pcs. Strawberries
- 2 tablespoons Olive Oil
- 1 teaspoon Coarse Salt – sea salt or Kosher salt

Process the strawberries in a blender or a food processor or simply mash with some utensils or your hands. Place the mashed strawberries in a bowl then add in the olive oil and the salt. Mix all the ingredients together to make a uniform substance, then massage onto your hands and your feet. Make sure to scrub gently or to massage onto the feet and hands to get the full effect. Leave it on for 10 minutes before rinsing off with some warm water then pat dry.

Skin-Like Buttermilk

Buttermilk, much like milk, also has beneficial effects on the skin. It contains lactic acid which exfoliates the skin to get rid of dry and dead skin cells. Simply soak a face cloth in cold buttermilk and leave it on dry or irritated skin for at least five minutes. Wash gently so that some of the lactic acid stays on your skin, and you can enjoy soft and smooth skin in just a matter of minutes.

Avocado Moisturizer

Avocados are great for the appetite, but even greater on the skin. The natural oils found in the fruit help to lubricate and moisten up the skin. Avocados are also rich in vitamins A, D, and E, which help to reduce fine lines and wrinkles. Simply mash some avocados and apply these to your body. Let it rest for ten to fifteen minutes, then rinse off with warm water.

Chapter 5: Natural Products, Safer Products

Now that you know that you can make beauty products at home, the only thing left to do is to actually make them. Some people may think that homemade products are unnecessary, especially if they do not buy too many products or treatments and if they are able to comfortably afford such products themselves. However, making these products at home is not all about the savings. Sure, you can save hundreds and even thousands of dollars every month if you go for homemade body treatments instead of the commercialized products, but there is so much more to natural products than you may think.

Giving your body a delightful treat doesn't have to be expensive, and neither does it have to be painful to the skin. People who use body products or any type of product on their skin should know that the body absorbs these products quickly and that the effects can be great. Applying these products can affect our appearance and our overall health as well, so these products should not be taken lightly. Unfortunately, majority of those who buy beauty products do not give their two cent's worth as to what the products actually contain or what the products are made of. As nice as it would be for all beauty product manufacturers to use only the best and safest ingredients possible, cost and other factors are leading them to put less-than-healthy ingredients into beauty products.

Making your own beauty products at home allows you to make sure that only healthy ingredients go into what you put on your body. The treatments provided in this book do not make use of any harsh chemicals or substances that could potentially damage the skin. Also, homemade treatments allow you to adjust your products according to your own preferences. If you find that a treatment is too strong, you can lessen the amount of acid. If the mixture is too rough or too dry, add a moisturizer to make it easier on the skin.

These homemade treatments are easy, fast, and affordable to do, and they are the healthiest treats that you can give your body.

Conclusion

Thank you again for purchasing this book!

I hope this book was able to help you understand the importance of treating your skin and body well and using only the best and natural ingredients for yourself.

The next step is to try out these homemade treatments and give yourself a treat! Take some out for yourself and spend a few minutes doing one of these treatments, then relax while you let the product take effect on you.

In addition, please remember to check out our Facebook page in order to find other resources and upcoming promotions:

https://www.facebook.com/joypublishing

With sincere thanks,

Scarlett O'Mara

One Last Thing...

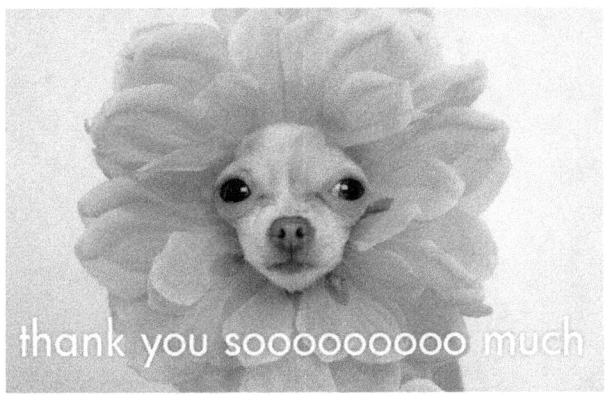

If you believe that this book is worth sharing, would you please take the time to let others know how it affected your life? If it turns out to make a difference in the lives of others, they will be forever grateful to you, as will I.

www.ingramcontent.com/pod-product-compliance
Lightning Source LLC
Chambersburg PA
CBHW070504290526
45790CB00003B/1091